I0423224

Healthy Without Chemicals

Treating common illnesses with acupressure and herbs

Nathalie Valkov PhD, L.Ac

ISBN -10: 1460977041
ISBN-13: 978-1460977040

Published by :
Nathalie Valkov PhD, L.Ac
4040 Civic Center Dr #200, San Rafael Ca 94903.
USA
818-230-2419, nvalkov@ttphc.com
ISBN-13: 978-1460977040
ISBN-10:1460977041

Cataloging-in-publication data

Valkov, Nathalie

Healthy Without Chemicals. Treating common
illnesses with acupressure and herbs/ Nathalie Valkov

ISBN-13:978-1460977040 ISBN-10:1460977041
1.   Health/Fitness 2. Alternative therapies

DISCLAIMER: The information given in this book has
been carefully researched. However, the author and
publisher cannot accept responsibility for any errors
or omission. They will not be held liable for any injury
or damages caused to the reader that may result from
the reader's acting upon and using the content of this
book. This book is intended to be purely informational
and is not meant to diagnose. Under no
circumstances does it replace the advice of a trained
medical practitioner.

I dedicate this book to my family.

My parents, Jean-Claude and Nicole Zambelli,

My two kids, Antoine and Julian,

My husband Emil,

My grand-mother, Raymonde Vinter,

and Sarah.

May they stay healthy and happy for all of eternity.

Foreword

In the last few years, I have seen more and more drugs being pulled off the market because they were killing people. As a practitioner of Asian Medicine, I treat my patients with natural remedies. But I am also well aware that many of you do not have access to the services I provide for my community. This book is therefore my attempt to bring you the tools you need to take a more proactive approach toward your own health. In many instances, chemicals are not necessary. Knowing that you may have other options is the first step in making informed decisions.

Table of content

67| Section II: Common illnesses

Introduction

Time is of the essence. If you bought this book, it is probably because you or someone you love may need a little bit of TLC. Some of you may be tired of taking pill after pill for ailments you may be able to treat yourself. For others, the pills may no longer be working. Regardless of the reasons why you bought this book, my guess is that you want the information to treat yourself and others, and you want it fast. I will therefore not bore you with the historical details and only give you a brief introduction summarizing the information relevant to the success of your treatment. For your convenience, I will also include, where advisable, possible Chinese herbal formulas that can be used for the condition being discussed.

What is acupressure?

Acupressure is an ancient traditional Asian medical modality. It is easy to perform and can be done anywhere. Generally one uses one or a few fingers, knuckles, or elbows to apply pressure to a specific area for 30 seconds to one minute. The areas where acupressure is applied are chosen based on acupuncture principles.

How does it work?

In traditional Asian medicine, pain or illness is caused by a blockage disrupting the flow of blood or energy to the affected area. Acupressure and acupuncture aim at removing this blockage by applying needles or pressure to points on the body known to regulate the flow of blood and energy to the area being treated.

According to Dr ichard Tan, another way of looking at this is by comparing your body to a switch board on which acupoints are the switches. By switching points on and off, you are sending your body messages on how to rebalance itself. It is, in my opinion, a very effective and clear way of explaining what acupressure does to be body.

Why do it?

First of all, it is free. It is something you can do for yourself that does not require medical insurance or paying someone's fees. Second, it is non-invasive. There is no insertion of any type of needle, no intake of any chemical. Third, you are in control. You choose when to do it, where to do it, and what pressure you do it at. You do not rely on anyone's schedule or expertise. Last but not least, you do it because if it does not help, it certainly will not hurt. And a lot of the time, it will actually help.

How to do it?

Again apply pressure to the chosen area following the instructions suggested in the subsequent pages for 30 seconds to one minute. Do not apply to much pressure. If it hurts, it is probably not doing you any good. You can also, if you choose, make a tiny circular motion right on the point.

Do not worry too much about having the right point location, as you will be using a finger (or a few) and the width of it will help you hit the point you want to reach. Furthermore, pictures with the location of the points you will need can be found in the back of section I for your convenience, as well as a description of where to find the points.

How the book is organized

After the introduction that you are reading right now you will find a quick and dirty look at oriental medicine. Reading it will not make your acupressure treatments better, but it is very basic information. The more curious readers should probably be referred to books such as "the web that has no weaver", a classic in oriental medicine.

Section I will cover point location. You will be given detailed descriptions of where the points are on the body, as well as pictures of their location on a model. The point location section is organized in numerical order for ease of access. It will also discuss basic technique of acupressure.

Section II will cover the different ailments I chose to discuss in this book. Each chapter will have a section with different signs and symptoms associated with the illness being discussed. It will describe the main characteristics of the disease. Then you will have a "point prescription" area that will only have a list of points to use during the treatment you planning to do. The "general" point prescription is to be used all the time. Modifications may appear under the "general" point prescription, but will be mentioned as such. These should only be done if the symptom associated with it is present. No description will be provided in this section as it was already described in section I. This is done to prevent tiresome repetitions as one point may be used for more than one illness. Finally you will find an "herbal advice" area where patent formulas that are reasonably easy to find are suggested where possible. For your convenience these formulas are written in bold.

A bit of advice

All that being said this book is not intended to self-diagnose or diagnose, and the intervention of a qualified health care professional for proper diagnosis and treatment is of the utmost importance. So if symptoms are severe or continue without improvement for a couple of days, please seek the advice of your medical doctor or acupuncturist/herbalist at once.

Warning

If you are pregnant, do not take herbs without checking with a knowledgeable health care professional first.

I also wanted to apologize in advance for any repetition that will be found in the book. They are intentional, but were not included in the text to bore you. As I must assume that most of my readers will not read this book cover to cover, some points need to be reiterated on different pages so they are not missed by the busy individual who will choose to concentrate on one ailment only. To all the other hard core acupressurists to be, I apologize.

Chapter 1:

A crash course in oriental medicine

Oriental medicine is composed of various methods of diagnosis and treatment that may include acupuncture, acupressure, moxa, cupping, herbs, qi gong exercises, diet, meditation, Tai Chi and/or life changes.

Oriental medicine is based on the assumption that our body relies on energy (Qi) that travels in a specific direction to function properly. Any blockage, redirection, decrease or excess storage of energy in a specific area of the body will cause an imbalance that may trigger a disease and possibly pain. These conditions may develop from toxic substances of the environment, poor nutrition, infectious diseases, overwork, overuse of a specific body part or organ, excessive exposure to heat, cold, damp, wind, or emotions.

Acupuncture and acupressure were developed thousands of years ago in China. Today, they are used in many parts of the world with great results. It is based on the theory that the insertion of needles or stimulation at specific points on the body will affect the patient's energy (either moving, tonifying, or draining) in order to restore balance and thus relieve patient's ailments.

Oriental medicine has been known to treat addictions, allergies, asthma, swellings, pains, arthritis, ADD/ADHD, digestive problems, hemorrhoids, immune system deficiency, insomnia, kidney problems, depression, anxiety, prostate problems, thyroid conditions, and many other ailments. It has also shown to be a great ally in the fight against cancer.

The goal of an acupuncture or acupressure treatment is to regulate the immune system, to alleviate pain or other debilitating symptoms and the balance the energy of the body to maximize the proper function of the body's organs.

An acupuncture treatment is generally not painful. The needles used are very thin and thus produce virtually no pain on insertion. Oftentimes, a sensation of well being is to be expected after the insertion is performed. An average treatment lasts about 30 minutes after needle insertion and may be accompanied by infrared heat therapy to increase the movement of Qi and to keep the patient comfortable. The number of treatment and the frequency at which treatments should be received depends on the person being treated, the nature of the problem, and the length of time the patient has been living with the issue. In China, people often get treated once a day for a few weeks or months. In the United States, very few people have the opportunity to get treated so often, so an average therapy will include one or two appointments a week for a few months.

Acupressure treatment should never be painful, and should be performed at least once a day but two or three times a day is even better. The effects will be milder than acupuncture but will produce results none the less, especially if used in conjunction with acupuncture treatment. As a matter of fact, it is very common for my patients to leave my office with an acupuncture chart where I mark all the points I would like them to do on themselves or have someone else perform on them until their next appointment. This not only helps prolong the effects of the acupuncture treatment, but it also involves the patient with his or her own recovery. By taking an active role in his or her treatment, he or she is sending the body a message that he or she is serious about getting better. By choosing the right points, he

17

or she lets the body know what needs to be fixed.

Acupressure is so effective, that on children, it often replaces acupuncture. For the little ones, electro-stimulation and laser stimulation may also be used. But regardless of the method of stimulation being used, the same points are always prescribed.

Herbal medicine is also a part of oriental medicine, and has also been practiced for thousands of years. Today, prescriptions are based on ancient formulas that have been time tested and that are known to have helped millions of people. The Chinese pharmacopoeia is comprised of hundreds of herbs, minerals and animal products that are combined to suit the constitution, the imbalance, and promote the immediate relief of symptoms of the individual being treated. Unfortunately, not all formulas are created equal. While most vendors provide access to very reliable formulas, others may not be as thorough. So before you buy your herbs, make sure the company that sells them is serious about getting you goods that do not contain heavy metals or pesticides. Even if the name of a formula is the same as another one, it does not mean that they came from the same source. Keep in mind however, that, when free of these pollutants and with the proper guidance, Chinese herbs can be very safe and effective.

Oriental medicine also encourages physical and mental exercises such as Qi Gong and mediation in order to promote the movement and generation (or gathering) of Qi. For instance, Qi Gong is a physical exercise that allows for very slow movement of the body along with breathing and visualization exercises.

Cupping refers to the use of suction cups to move Qi and blood to alleviate pain, stimulate organ functions, and regulate the immune system. It has been known to not only reduce pain, but also alleviate coughing and stopping asthma attacks.

Moxa refers to the use of mugwort. The herb is burned close to or on a specific acupuncture point to stimulate that point, warm the body, or simply to tonify the body in general.

Acupuncture, acupressure, herbal therapy, moxa, cupping, Qi Gong and meditation may be prescribed in combination or separate from one another, depending on the person's imbalances and constitution. They, however, all have the goal of restoring balance and harmony to the patient being treated.

Section I

Point

location

I have chosen to give you the point locations for the points used during the treatment first so you could familiarize yourself with their names and numbers. I do not suggest that you pour over the rather long list of points in details at this point as you would probably be quickly overwhelmed by the dryness of the information provided. You will have plenty of time in the future to go back to the points you need for your treatment when you need them.

If you feel the location description is not anatomical enough for you, please feel free to consult *Chinese Acupuncture and Moxibustion* as I am aware that my attempt at simplicity may not please the more purist readers. Also keep in mind the pictures that follow the descriptions will be an invaluable help to find the point.

Note: when referring to a finger width, I am generally referring to you thumb.

Lung meridian

LU1: About 2 finger widths below the collar bone at the edge of the shoulder muscle.

LU5: At the elbow crease on the outer side of the big tendon that can be felt when the elbow is slightly bent.

LU7: On the side of the wrist/arm, thumb side, about 2 finger width from the base of the thumb, in the depression.

LU9: On the wrist crease, palm side, aligned with the base of the thumb, just on the outside of where you take your pulse (where you feel a pulse)

LU10: On the palmar side, halfway between the base of the thumb and the wrist crease at the junction of where the skin changes color.

LU11: Very close to the thumb nail corner closest to the inside of the body when the palm of the hands are resting on the knees.

Large intestine meridian

LI4: On the back of the hand, between the thumb and the index finger. When the thumb and the index finger are held together, apiece of flesh appears. This is the general area of where you want to be.

LI11: On the inner arm, between the end of the elbow crease and the funny bone toward the outside of the body.

LI20: On the outside of the nostrils almost level with the lower part of the ears.

Spleen meridian

SP6: About 3 thumb width up the leg from the bone present on the inner ankle, just to the back of the bone that can be felt in the inner leg

SP9: Going all the way up the leg from the bone on the inside of the ankle, the point is in a depression just below the bone that makes up part of the knee.

SP10: About 2 thumb width above the knee bulge toward the central side of the leg.

SP21: Under the armpit, on the line going from the center of the armpit and straight down, slightly below the line drawn horizontally from the nipple.

Stomach meridian

ST2: When looking straight forward, the point is directly below the pupil (black circle in the center of the eye), about one to half finger width from the edge of the bone just below the eyeball. When touching the area, you should feel a little hole.

ST8: Just behind the hairline, from the midline of the forehead, measure a whole width of your hand (the knuckle part) toward the outside of the body.

ST9: Level with the tip of the Adam's apple, about mid neck, about 2 finger widths toward the outside of the body.

ST25: About 2 finger widths toward the outside of the body, level with the belly button.

ST36: 3 finger widths below the lower part of the knee, about one finger width from the bone toward the outside of the body

ST37: 6 finger widths below the lower part of the knee, about one finger width from the bone toward the outside of the body

ST40: 8 finger widths below the lower part of the knee, about two finger width from the bone toward the outside of the body

ST44: Between the 2nd and 3rd toe, the big toe being the 1st toe, just where the toes end and the foot begins.

Heart meridian

HT7: On the palmer side, at the pinky end of the wrist crease.

HT8: On the palm, on the line starting between the pinky and the 4th finger toward the wrist crease. Make a fist and the tip of the pinky rests on the point.

Small intestine meridian

SI3: Make a fist. You will find the point on the side of the pinky, just behind the knuckle bone going toward the wrist where the skin changes color.

SI14: From the base of the neck, go down the spine about 2 finger width then 3 finger widths toward the outside of the body.

SI15: From the base of the neck at the spine, go 2 finger widths toward the outside of the body.

Kidney meridian

KID1: At the bottom of the foot, divide the sole in 3. The first division starts at the toes. Go to the end of the first division (toward the heel) and find the point at the center of the foot. Another way of finding it is to point your toes. The point is in the depression that forms on the sole of the food.

KID3: The point is between the bone on the inside of the ankle and the Achilles' tendon, level with the tip of the bone.

KID7: Go between the bone on the inside of the ankle and the Achilles' tendon, then go up 2 finger widths, staying in front of the Achilles' tendon.

Note: Kidney points appear on the pictures with the notation KI instead of KID

Urinary bladder meridian

UB1: Just to the outside and slightly above the inner corner the eye.

UB10: On the back of the head, about 1.5 thumb width from the midline, slightly below the base of the skull.

UB11: On the upper back, level with the upper border of the shoulder blade, about 1.5 thumb width away from the spine.

UB13: On the upper back, about 1/3 of the way down from the upper border to the bottom of the shoulder blade , about 1.5 thumb width away from the spine.

UB15: On the back, about midway from the upper border to the bottom of the shoulder blade, about 1.5 thumb width away from the spine.

UB17: On the back, level with the bottom of the shoulder blade, about 1.5 thumb width away from the spine.

UB18: On the back, about a ¼ of the distance from UB17 to UB23 down from UB17, 1.5 thumb width away from the spine

UB19: On the back, slightly above the midway point between UB17 and UB23, 1.5 thumb width away from the spine

UB20: On the back, slightly below the midway point between UB17 and UB23, 1.5 thumb width away from the spine.

UB21: On the back, about a ¼ of the distance from UB17 to UB23, up from UB23 and 1.5 thumb widths away from the spine.

UB23: At waist level, about 1.5 thumb width away from the spine.

UB40: At the back of the knee, on the crease, midway between the two tendons.

UB60: On the outside of the ankle, between the pointy tip and the Achilles tendon.

UB62: On the outside of ankle, just below and half a thumb width from point tip of the ankle.

UB67: On the outside of the little toe, at the outside corner of the nail, closest to the body.

Note: Urinary Bladder points appear on the pictures with the notation BL instead of UB.

Pericardium meridian

PC5: On the inner aspect of the forearm (palm side), about 3 thumb widths up from the wrist crease at the midline.

PC6: On the inner aspect of the forearm (palm side), about 2 thumb widths up from the wrist crease at the midline.

PC7: At the wrist crease (palm side), in the middle.

PC9: Feel good point. In the center of the tip of the middle finger.

San Jiao meridian

SJ5: Opposite to PC6. On the outer aspect of the forearm, 2 thumb widths up from the wrist crease, in a depression between the two bones (in the middle).

SJ6: Opposite to PC5. On the outer aspect of the forearm, 3 thumb widths up from the wrist crease, in a depression between the two bones (in the middle).

Liver meridian

LIV2: On the top of the foot, between the first and second toe, about ½ a thumb width from the edge of the web, toward the body.

LIV3: On top of the foot, moving toward the body between the first and second toe, LIV3 is in the first hollow.

Gallbladder meridian

GB2: In front of the ear, in the hollow that can be felt when the month is open.

GB5: About half way from the front corner of the head to the top of the ear.

GB13: At the intersection of the line going up from the outer corner of the eye and half a thumb width from the hairline.

GB14: On the forehead, 1 thumb width above the eye brow, directly above the pupil when the eyes are looking straight forward.

GB20: At the base of the skull in the first hollow as you move away from the spine. It is generally the most tender point in the area.

GB21: Halfway between the spine in the neck and the tip of the shoulder, at the highest part of the muscle found on top of the shoulder.

GB34: Below the side of the knee, in the hollow just between the bone.

GB37: On the outside of the leg, 5 thumb widths going up following the bone from the pointy tip of the ankle.

GB41: On the top of the foot, between the bones that extend from the fourth and the little toe, in the depression closest to the body.

Ren meridian

Ren3: On the midline in the front of the body, 4 thumb widths down from the belly button.

Ren4: On the midline in the front of the body, 3 thumb widths down from the belly button.

Ren6: On the front midline of the body, 1.5 thumb widths down from the belly button.

Ren12: On the midline in the front of the body, 4 thumb widths up from the belly button.

Ren13: On the midline in the front of the body, 5 thumb widths up from the belly button.

Ren14: On the midline in the front of the body, 6 thumb widths up from the belly button.

Ren17: On the front midline of the body, between the nipples.

Ren22: On the midline in the front of the body, at the lower end of the throat, just above the breast bone. This point should only receive very light acupressure.

Du meridian

DU4: On the midline of the lower back, on the spine, level with the waist.

DU14: On the midline, in the back at the base of the neck, level with the upper border of the shoulder blade.

DU20: On top of the head, at the intersection between the line going straight up from the tip of the ears and that going from the tip of the nose.

DU23: At the top of the head on the midline, 1 thumb width behind the front hairline.

DU24: At the top of the head on the midline, ½ a thumb width behind the front hairline.

Extra and ear points

Anmian: Behind the lower third of the ear.

Bitong: At the lowest point of the bone on the side of the nose.

Dingchuan: half to one thumb width from DU14

Ear Shen men: Ear point. In the back of the small, triangular depression at the front top of the ear.

Qiu Hou: along the lower border of the eye socket, ¾ of the way from the inner corner of the eye to the outer corner. Only light pressure should be used when going acupressure on this point.

Taiyang: At the temple, in the depression about one thumb width back of the midpoint between the outer extremity of the eyebrow and the outer corner of the eye.

Yao Tong Xue: On the back of the hand, two points located between the bone extensions of the second and third finger, and fourth and fifth finger. In the depression closest to the body.

Yao Yan: At the dimples on the lower back about 3.5 thumb widths from the spine.

Yintang: midpoint between the eyebrows.

Yu Yao: In the center of the eyebrow.

Acupressure techniques

There are two acupressure techniques that I like using and teaching.

The first one is easy, and does not require any special skills. It is the first one I learned and I still occasionally practice it. It only requires locating the point. Then using your thumb or your three middle fingers, massage the point by applying a circular motion for 30 seconds to a minute on children, and one to two minutes on adults. A moderate amount of pressure should be applied, and the treatment should, in my opinion, be painless.

The second method is very easy on the practitioner's joints and quite effective on the person being treated. The three middle fingers should be applied to the point with only very mild pressure. The pressure should be maintained until a sense of balance is attained. Concretely, this would translate into feeling rhythmic pulsations in one's fingers. Two points may be done at the same time.

When a point can be found on both sides of the body, it is best to apply the acupressure to both sides. But when in a hurry, do the acupressure on one arm and then on the opposite leg.

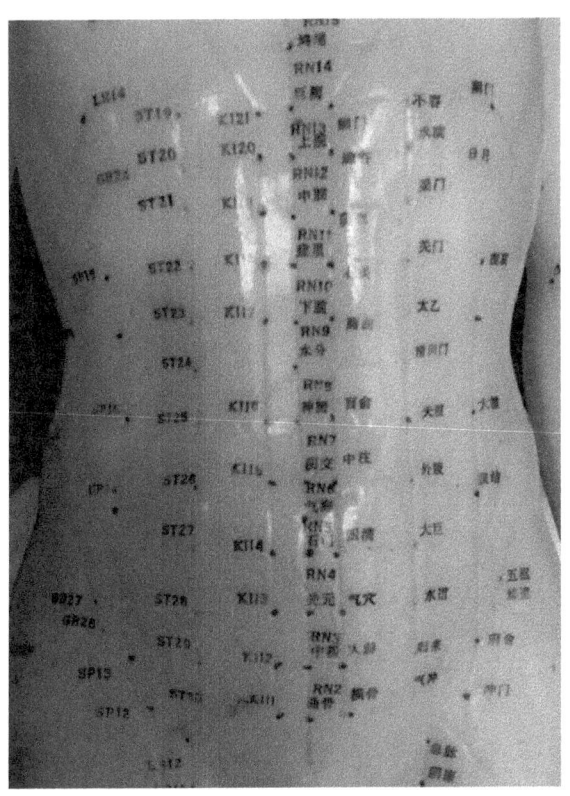

Photo 1. Torso

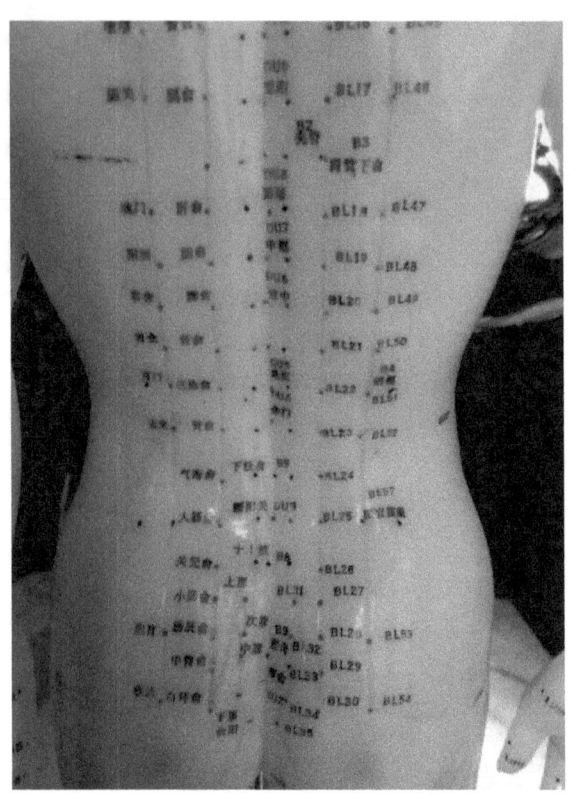

Picture 2. Back

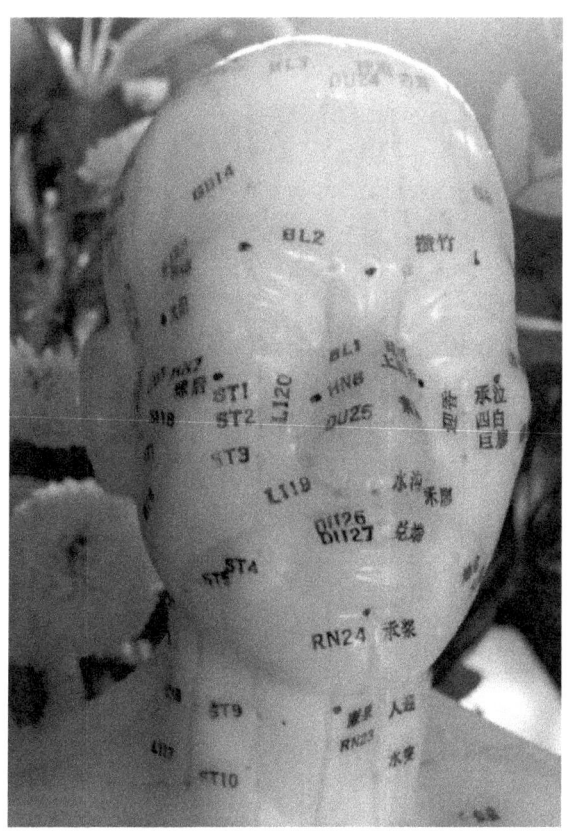

Picture 3. Face

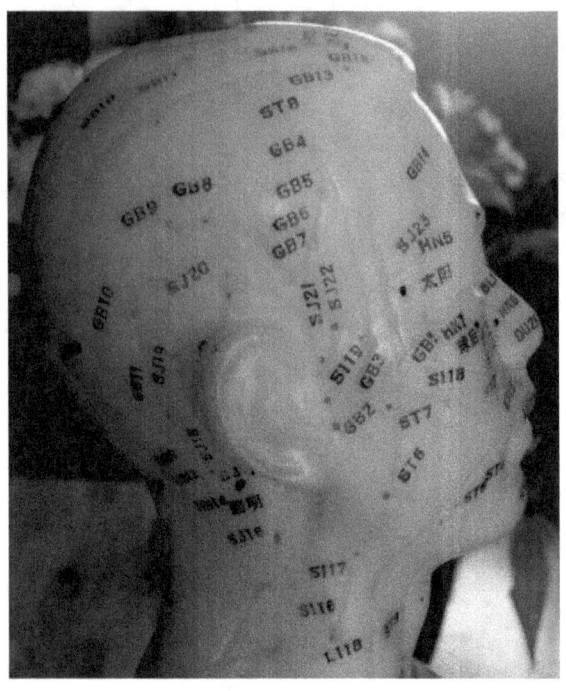

Picture 4. Side of head

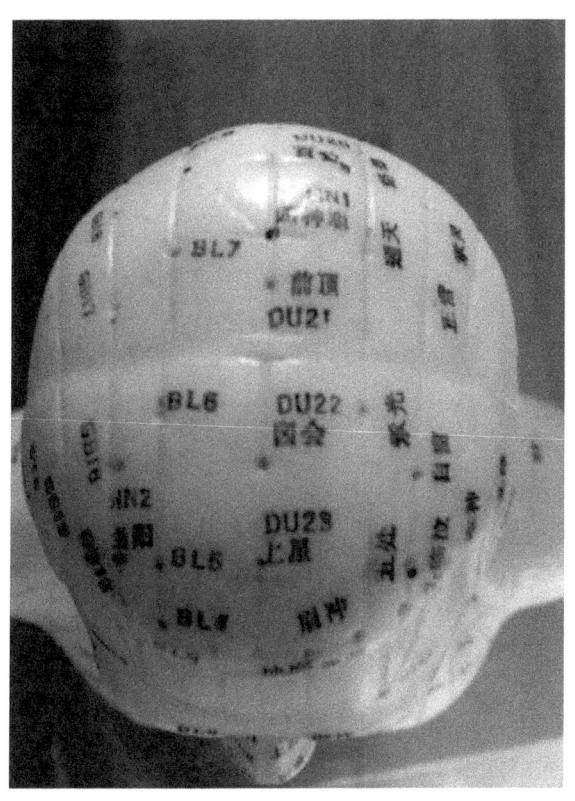

Picture 5. Top of head

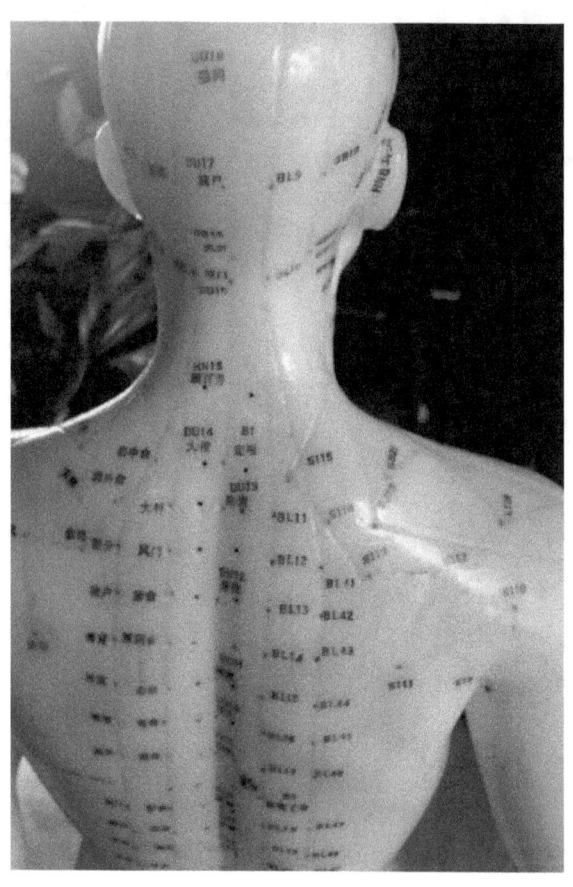

Picture 6. Upper back and back of head

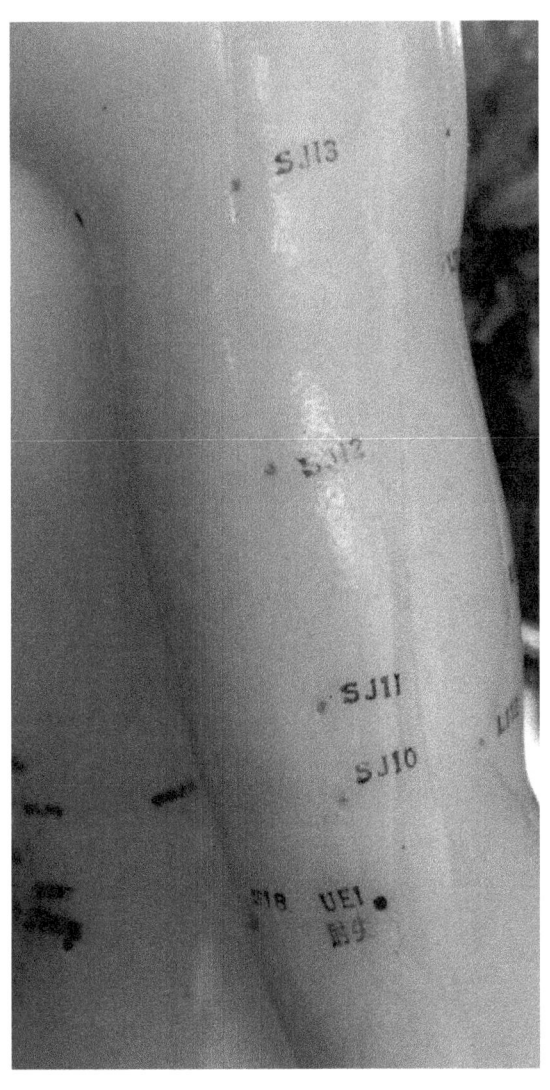

Picture 7. Back of arm (outer portion)

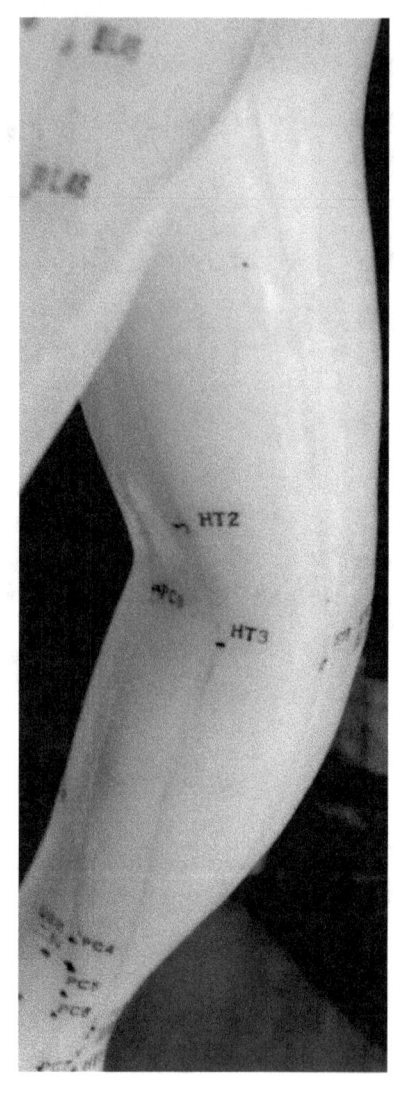

Picture 8. Back of arm (inner portion)

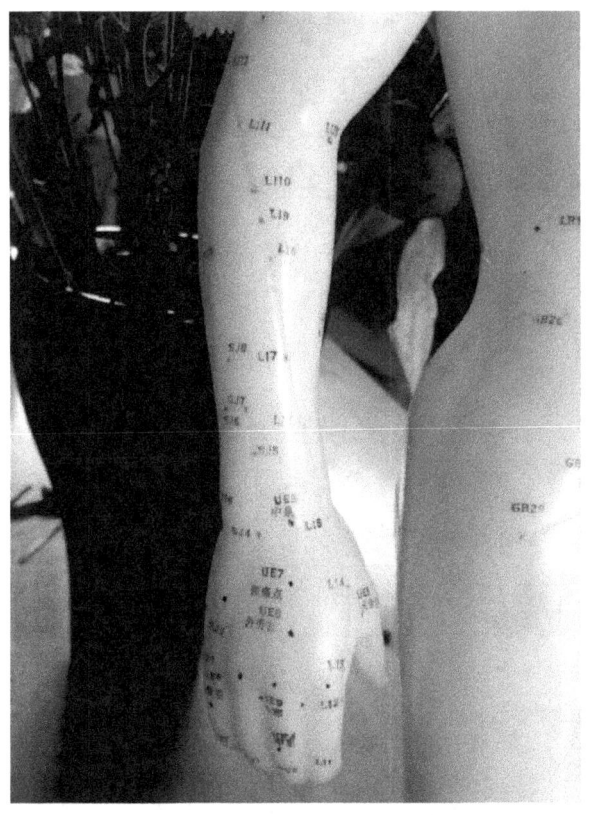

Picture 9. Forearm

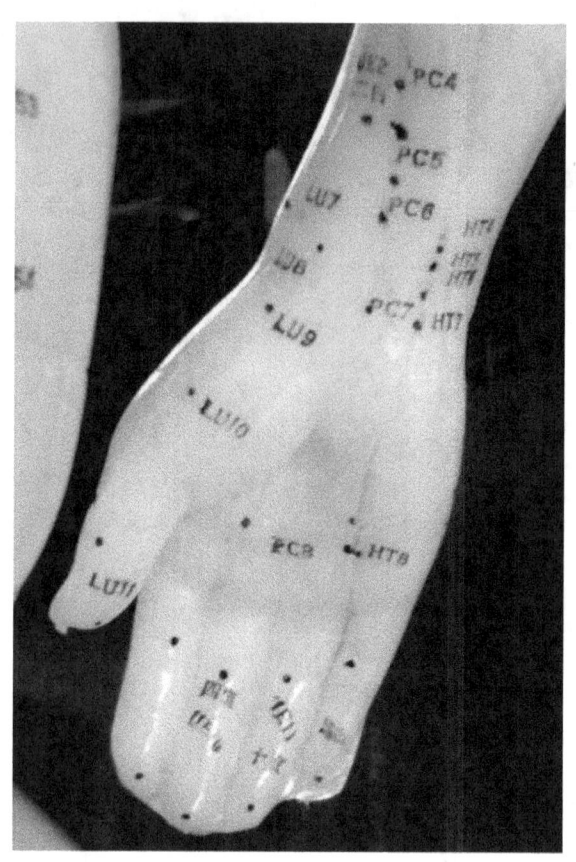

Picture 10. Palm

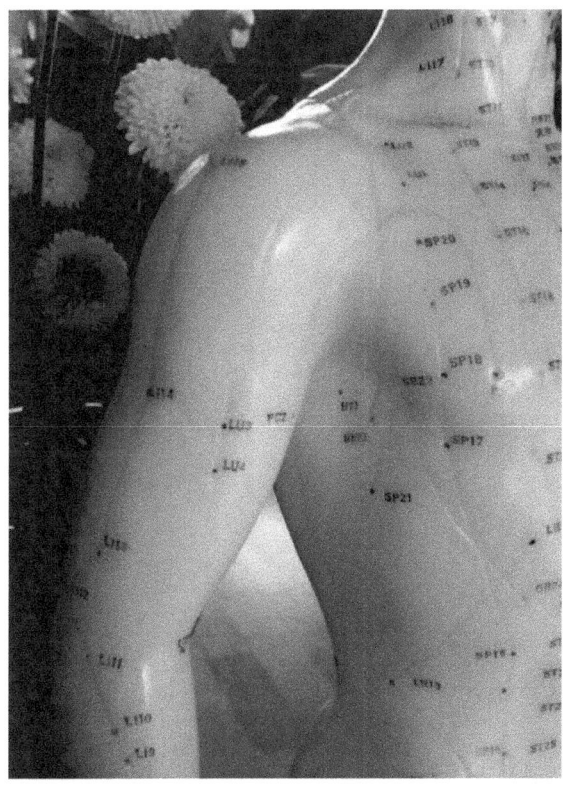

Picture 11. Upper arm and side of torso

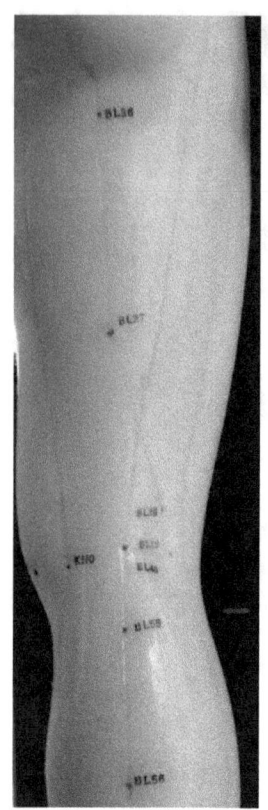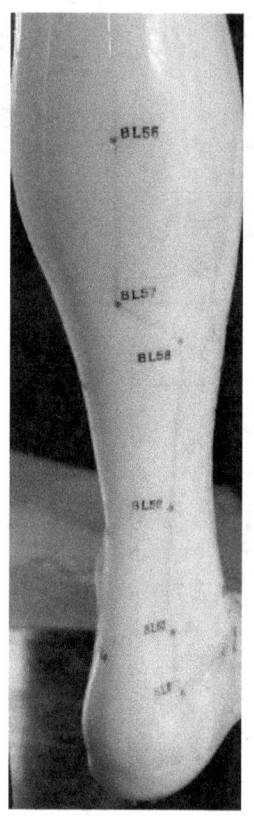

Picture 12 and 13. Upper and lower back leg.

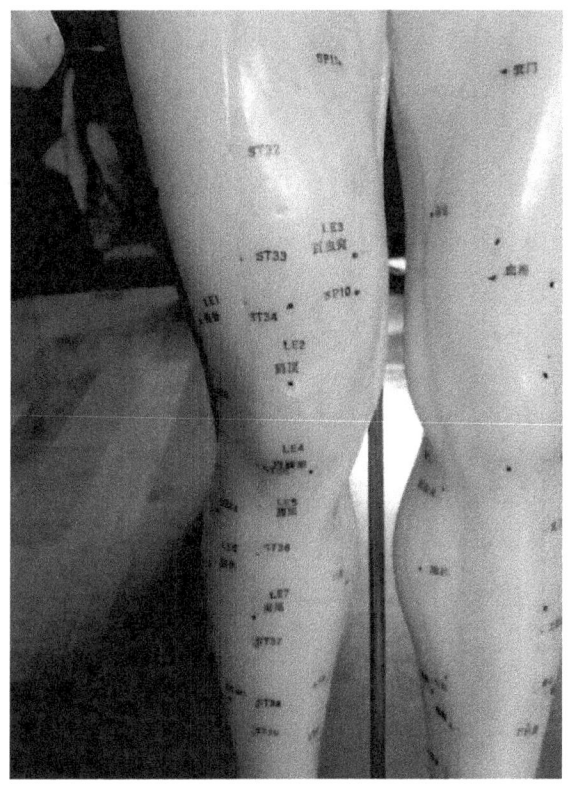

Picture 14. Front legs

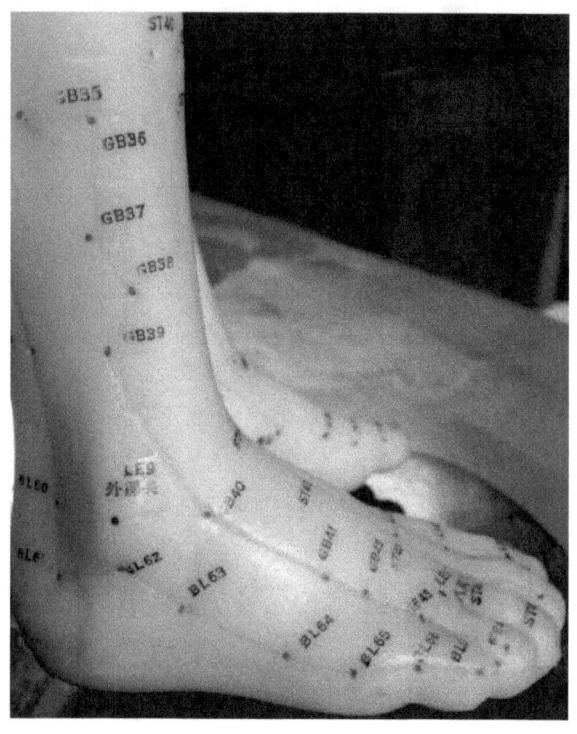

Picture 15. Outer ankle and foot

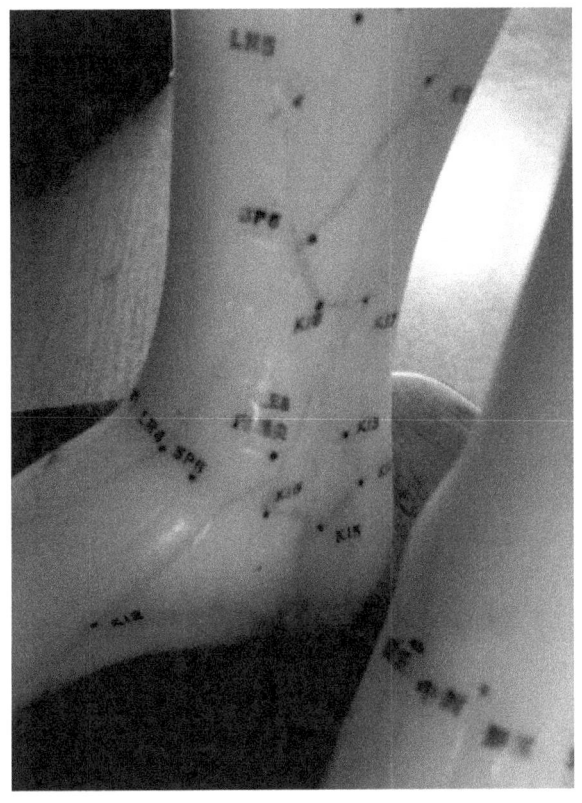

Pictures 16. Inner side of ankle and foot

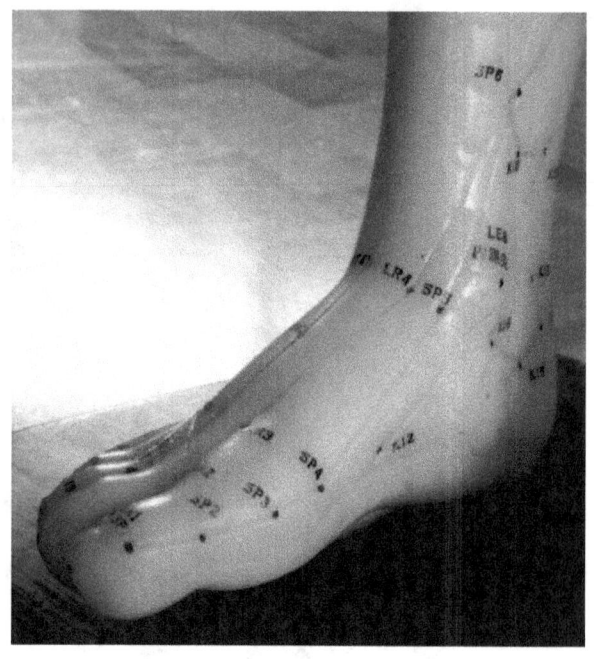

Picture 17. Foot

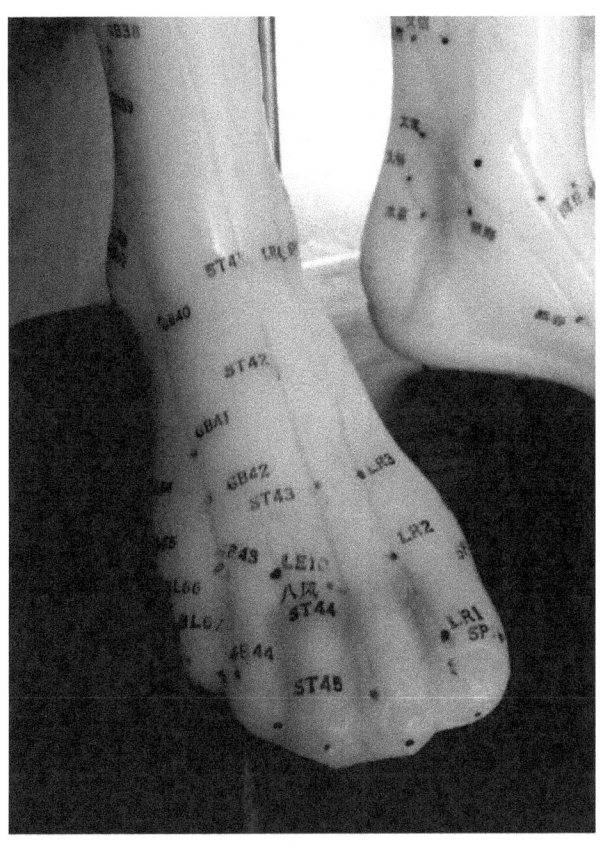

Pictures 18. Foot

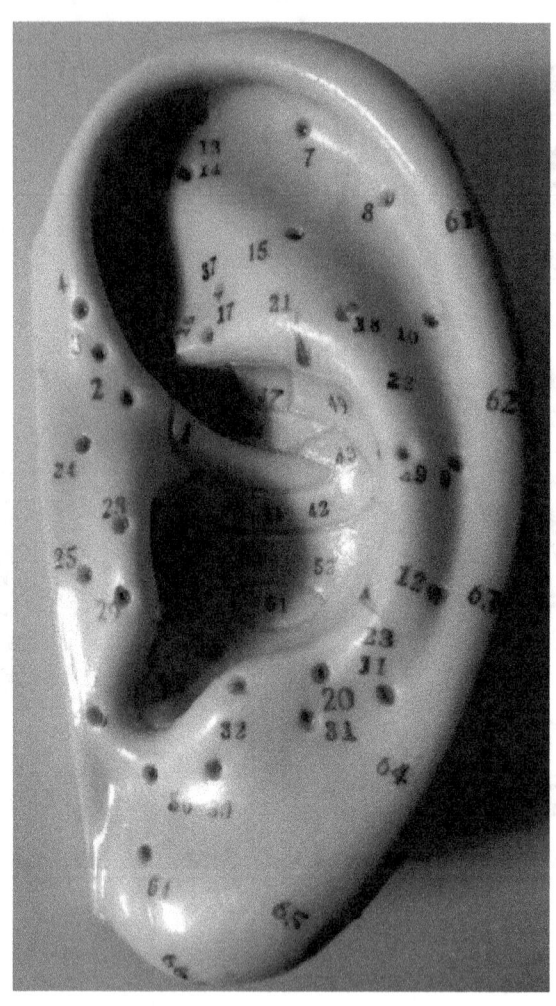

Picture 19. Ear

Section II

Common

illnesses

Chapter 2:

Common Cold

Signs and symptoms

Colds generally do not involve fever (only low grade- below 100 if present) or headaches. Only mild general aches and pains may be present with minimal fatigue and weakness. A stuffy or runny nose with possible sinus pressure and sore throat are very common. Sneezing is usually present as well. There may also be a hacking cough with relatively large amounts of sputum coming up.

Point prescription

General: UB13, LU1, ST36, LU7, LI4, DU14, SJ5, GB20

Stuffy nose: LI20 or bitong

Sore throat: LU10, LU11*

*When doing acupressure on LU11 for sore throat, use your nail to dig into the skin. Do not break the skin or attempt to get blood.

Herbal advice

In the very early stages of colds, when the symptoms are first being noticed, start taking **Gan Mao Ling** immediately. The dosage indicated on the box/bottle may not be appropriate for your weight, so please call your local acupuncturist or the number listed in the back of our book for dosage advice. Gan Mao Ling may also be taken preventatively when you are around people with cold. This will decrease your chances of developing symptoms. For cough a **loquat and fritillary extract** syrup can be taken.

Note: In adult patients I have prescribed as much Gan Mao Ling as 12 pills every 4 hours until symptoms disappear and then 8 pills 3 times daily for two more days. However, this amount was prescribed under close supervision.

Chapter 3:

Flu

Signs and symptoms

The flu is characterized by a fever of over 100F that typically lasts 3 to 4 days. Headaches, along with general body aches and pains are very common and often severe. Fatigue and weakness can be present for as long as 3 weeks, and extreme exhaustion is felt in the first few days. Occasional stuffy nose, sore throat and sneezing can be seen. Chest discomfort and a dry nonproductive cough can be present as well. Beware: a poorly treated flu can turn into bronchitis or even pneumonia which will require immediate medical attention.

Point prescription

General: LU10, LU5, DU14, SJ5, LI11, ST36

Sore throat: LU11

Heavy chest and pain: PC6, Ren17, SJ6

Cough: LU7, Ren22

Lots of yellow mucus: ST40, SP9

Herbal advice

In the very early stages of the flu, when the symptoms are first being noticed, start taking **Gan Mao Ling** immediately.

The dosage indicated on the box may not be enough, so please call your local acupuncturist or the number listed in the back of our book for dosage advice. Gan Mao Ling may also be taken preventatively when you are around people with the flu. This will decrease your chances of developing symptoms.

Note: In adult patients I have prescribed as much Gan Mao Ling as 12 pills every 4 hours until symptoms disappear and then 8 pills 3 times daily for two more days. However, this amount was prescribed under close supervision.

Chapter 4:

Stomach Flu (gastroenteritis)

Signs and symptoms

Signs and symptoms may be similar to the flu but nausea, vomiting, abdominal discomfort and diarrhea may be present as well. The same caution described for the flu should be observed for the stomach flu. Beware: if the pain starts before the vomiting, you may be suffering from appendicitis and may require immediate medical attention.

Point prescription

General: ST25, ST36, ST37, Ren14, Ren13, Ren4, LI4, LI11

Nausea and vomiting: PC6

Diarrhea: ST44, SP9

Herbal advice

Curing pills can be taken any time after the onset of symptoms. The pills will help with the nausea, vomiting, abdominal discomfort and diarrhea. For details on how many pills to take and the frequency at which to take them please contact your acupuncturist or call the number listed at the back of the book.

Note: More often than not, the dosage on the bottle is not enough for us big boned Americans. I have prescribed as much as 5 pills every 4 hours until symptoms subside. But as with everything else the dosage requirement is weight related, so the advice of an herbalist is strongly suggested.

Chapter 5:

Asthma

Signs and symptoms

The acute phase of an asthma attack is characterized by wheezing, shortness of breath, cough, difficult breathing. In the chronic phase, symptoms are not as obvious. Constant mild wheezing, fatigue and shortness of breath will be present.

Asthma is a very serious and potentially life threatening condition. It is not advised to rely solely on acupressure to treat this condition. This treatment modality can help lessen some of the symptoms during an acute phase, but being under the care of a health care professional is essential. During the chronic phase, acupressure can help reduce the symptoms and decrease the number of asthma attacks.

Point prescription

Acute phase general: Dingchuan, Ren22, Ren17, LU7, LI4, LU5, ST40, SP9

Chronic phase general: UB13, UB20, UB23, LU9, ST36, SP9, ST40, SP6, KID3, Ren17, Ren12, Ren4

Herbal Advice

Treatment of asthma in the acute phase is possible with the help of a qualified healthcare professional, namely a licensed acupuncturist. Self-medication is not advisable. During the chronic phase **Yu Ping Feng San** and **concentrated royal jelly capsules** may be taken to strengthen the body and help prevent or lessen further attacks.

Chapter 6:

Headaches

Signs and symptoms

Tension headache: generally start at the back of the neck or the base of the skull and work their way up toward the front of the head. They tend to occur on both sides and even though they are rarely a daily occurrence they can happen every day. These types of headaches are rarely accompanied by nausea or sensitivity to light and sound, and are generally mild.

Migraine headaches: intense pain usually on one side of the head and alternating sides from one attack to the next. If the pain is consistently on the same side, please consult a medical doctor to rule out any other serious illnesses. Nausea, vomiting, visual disturbances and sensitivity to light and sound are very common with this type of headache.

Cluster headaches: these headaches occur sometimes more than once a day, every day, for weeks or months. They generally last between 30 and 90 minutes and are characterized by a severe pain behind one eye. Attacks generally occur at the same time every day and may wake a person up from a deep sleep.

Point prescription

General: LI4, GB20, SP6, UB18, UB20, UB23, ST36

Headache in front of head: ST8, Yintang, ST44, DU24, GB14

Headache on top of head: DU20, SI3, LIV3, UB67

Headache in back of head: UB60, SI3

Headache on side of head: Taiyang, GB41, GB5

With nausea: PC6

Pain behind the eye: UB1, ST2, Qiu Hou, GB2, Yu Yao

Herbal advice

A combination of **Migratrol** and **herbal analgesic** from Evergreen herbs over a day or two generally takes care of the pain. The only problem is that these products can only be found at a health care professional's office. For help with obtaining these products, please call the number given at the back of the book or email me directly at nvalkov@ttphc.com.

Chapter 7:

Depression

Signs and symptoms

They include profound sadness, loss of interest in daily or favorite activities, feelings of worthlessness or guilt, feeling of emptiness, trouble making decisions, thoughts of suicide or death, fatigue, sleep disturbance, increased or decreased appetite, difficult concentration, body aches and pain. Not all symptoms need to be present to be diagnosed with depression. It is my opinion that people suffering from depression should be under the care of a mental health professional. However it is also my opinion and experience that people suffering from this illness should seriously consider acupuncture and the use of Chinese herbs before they start taking pharmaceuticals. With proper guidance, depression sufferers can get off their medication and use herbs to combat this devastating disease. Acupressure in this case will help reduce the severity of symptoms and prolong the effect of acupuncture treatment.

Point prescription

General: DU24, GB13, Ren17, LI4, LIV3, ST36, PC6

Short temper and irritability: LIV2, GB34

Crying spells: HT7, SP6

Herbal advice

Chai Hu Shu Gan San can be used to resolve the imbalances that cause depression. However, when the person being treated cries a lot, **Gan Mai Da Zao Tang** may a better choice. If these do not relieve symptoms within two weeks or if symptoms are severe please consult a licensed acupuncturist and a mental health professional at once.

Chapter 8:

Stress

Signs and symptoms

Stress affects all aspects of your being. What is a normal response by your body to an outside stimulus can become detrimental to your health if it is sustained for too long. Signs and symptoms can be both mental and physical. They include neck and shoulder pain, low back soreness, occasional headaches, alternating diarrhea and constipation, weight issues, skin outbreaks, loss of sex drive, sleep disorders, teeth grinding, memory loss, difficulty making decisions, over thinking, anxiety, irritability, and more. Some of these symptoms may also be part of other more serious issues that may need to be ruled out by a health care professional. Once this has been done, acupressure can be quite effective at relieving stress.

Point prescription

General: DU24, Ear shen men, Ren17, LI4, LIV3, PC6

Shoulder pain: GB21, SI15, SI14

Neck tension: GB20, UB10, UB11

Low back problems: UB23, Yaoyan, UB40, UB62, Yaotongxue

Herbal advice

Xiao Chai Hu Tang can be taken to help alleviate the symptoms associated with stress and to help better cope with everyday life.

Chapter 9:

Hypertension

Signs and symptoms

Many people have no symptoms per say and need the input of a health care professional that will test them to diagnose. A simple machine can also be bought in pharmacies and drug stores, but they are less reliable than the instruments your health care professional will use. Individuals are considered to have hypertension when their blood pressure is higher than 140/90. That being said, there are some warning signs that may give you an indication that you need to be seen by your primary care provider. They include headaches, particularly in the morning, confusion, dizziness, and ringing in the ear.

Point prescription

General: ST9 (massage gently in a downward motion), LI4, LIV3, DU20, ST36, KID1, UB17, UB18, UB19, UB20.

With headache: see the headache section of the book.

With dizziness: KID3, LIV2, ST40, SP6.

Herbal advice

One of the useful formulas used in Chinese medicine is **Tian Ma Gou Teng**

Yin. However, hypertension is difficult to treat and may require the intervention of a licensed acupuncturist who will be able to customize your formula to match your needs. You can also increase your consumption of fresh raw vegetable and fruit while cutting down on salt and salty foods like soy sauce. **Garlic** is also effective in lowering blood pressure.

Chapter 10:

Allergies (Hay fever)

Signs and symptoms

In general you will suffer from one or more of these symptoms seasonally: sneezing, runny nose, nasal congestion, body itching, itchy red eyes, itchy throat, post nasal drip, headache in the front of the head. You may also have these symptoms all year long if they are associated with things like fungus, dust and animal dander.

Point prescription

General: LI20, Yintang, LI4, DU23, UB13, ST36

With severe stuffy nose: Bitong

With coughing: LU7

With lots of mucus and phlegm: ST40

Herbal advice

Bi Yan Pian is a good formula to use for a stuffy or runny nose, or other symptoms due to allergies. However when coughing is present this formula will not be sufficient and a trip to your acupuncturist may be necessary. If you do not have access to one, you may call our office at the number listed in the back of the book or go to www.DiabetesOrNot.com.

Chapter 11:

Insomnia

Signs and symptoms

Insomnia may be described in a few different ways. It can be experienced as the difficulty to fall asleep, or the inability to stay asleep in the early morning. It may also be that you are waking up many times during the night or that you wake up tired due to a restless night. Either way, it is insomnia and it can cause undesired consequences such a fatigue, excessive sleepiness during the day, difficulty focusing or irritability to only name a few.

Point prescription

General: Anmian, HT7, PC6, SP6, UB18, UB19, UB20, UB21, UB23, ST36, Ear shenmen, DU20

Herbal advice

You can take **An Mien Pien** to help with your insomnia, but unlike western medication the effects may be seen a few days or even an few weeks after you start taking your herbs. Since Chinese medicine is interested in treating the cause of a disease, it may take longer than the western drugs. But the Chinese formulas are non-habit forming and will actually help you to become medication free in the future. If this formula is not strong enough, stronger ones can be designed for you by an oriental medical practitioner.

The foods you eat can also help you go to sleep. Foods that are high in tryptofan will help you sleep. They include turkey, tuna, figs, banana, yogurt, and milk (warm with honey is even better). Other foods such as tomatoes, eggplant, potatoes, spinach, avocados, oranges, pineapples, grape, coffee, tea, chocolate, cheese, ham, bacon and sausages can have the opposite effect. So try and stay away from them after lunch.

A warm bath just before bedtime may also be helpful with a few drops of lavender essential oil.

Chapter 12:

Diabetes

Signs and symptoms

Diabetes is a very serious illness that requires sustained medical attention to ensure proper treatment. You may not have any symptoms and still have this disease. The complications include heart problems, eye problems, kidney problems that will have a terribly negative impact on your way of life if it does not kill you.

But here is what you can do to prevent complications. Have a yearly checkup to make sure your blood sugar level is normal. If you already have been diagnosed with the disease follow your health care provider's instructions. If you are very thirsty, have to pee often, have unusual weight loss, increased fatigue, feel irritable or have blurry vision, you should consider going to the health care practitioner for proper diagnosing.

Acupressure and herbs can help reduce the amount of western medication you need. In mild cases you may even be able to stay away from drugs altogether provided you follow the proper diet. But blood sugars should always be checked regularly to be sure that they are returning to normal range and staying there.

Chapter 13:

Impotence (erectile dysfunction)

Signs and symptoms

Erectile dysfunction is the recurring inability to sustain an erection long enough to have sex, and/or the inability to ejaculate. The incidence of such occurrence increases with age, and many men suffer in silence from this affliction, too embarrassed to discuss it with anyone. It is very common in the over 60 population, and many sufferers turn to products such as Viagra for help. However, risks associated with such product are not negligible and alternatives such as acupressure and herbs have got to be better for your health than those. Keep in mind that acupressure and herbs are not a quick fix and that it may take a few months of consistent treatment to start seeing improvement. So be patient.

Point prescription

General: UB23, UB15, DU4, KID3, KID7, SP6, SP9, ST36, Ren3, Ren4, Ren6, HT7

Herbal advice

A combination of Wu Zi Yan Zong Wan and Gui Pi Wan may be enough to help with this issue. But treatment should be following for a few months before evaluating its efficacy. As mentioned in the previous chapter, Cordyceps sinensis is a good adjunct for this treatment.

Chapter 14:

Irritable Bowel Syndrome

Signs and symptoms

Symptoms change from person to person. You can feel abdominal pain (stomach ache) constantly or it may come and go. The pain should go away when you go to the bathroom to have a bowel movement. There may be changes in the number of times you go per day and the look and shape of the stool. You may have diarrhea or constipation, or both may be alternating. You may have difficulty going. You may feel you have to go right away, or even feel like you are not done when you actually are. You may feel bloated and gassy. You may also suffer from anxiety, depression, sleep and/or bladder problems, head and/ or backache, fatigue, lower sex drive or pain during intercourse, or palpitations. Generally, stress and meals makes things worse. Doctors consider that these symptoms should last at least 12 weeks before you are diagnosed with this syndrome.

If your symptoms are getting worse and the pain is not relieved by going to the bathroom or passing gas, feel less anger, more tiredness than usual, losing weight without trying, can pinpoint the pain to a specific area or see blood in your stool, please contact your health care professional at once.

Point prescription

General: Ren12, Ren6, ST25, SP6, ST36, LIV3, LI4

Herbal advice

Shu Gan Wan may be a good choice of patent formula to help with this problem, but it will not cover all cases. If a feeling of incomplete bowel movement is present **Wu Mei Wan** may be a better choice. The best option is **GI Harmony** from Evergreen herbs but it is not easily found.

Chapter 15:
Fibromyalgia

Signs and symptoms

Symptoms include neck, shoulder, back, arms and leg pain, more specifically in muscles, tendons, and ligaments. There can also be muscle tenderness which may be worse in the morning, soreness, aching, and numbness. Unlike arthritis, the joints are not affected. It may also be difficult to sleep. There may be stiffness, fatigue, headaches, irregular bowel movements, inability to concentrate, loss of memory, and depression.

Point prescription

General: LI4, LIV3, PC6, SJ5, ST36, SP21, Ren12, ST25, Ren6, SP6, SP9, ST44

With severe fatigue: Ren4

With stabbing pain: PC5, SP10

Herbal advice

Xiao Yao San is the first formula that should be taken, along with Ban Xia Xie Xin Tang with loose stools or diarrhea, and Bu Zhong Yi Qi Tang for fatigue. Fibromyalgia may have many faces. The best thing to do is to consult first with a licensed acupuncturist for the appropriate formula and to use this book for enhancement of treatment.

Chapter 16:

Conclusion

In this book I have discussed the symptoms, point prescriptions, point location, and possible herbal treatment for quite a few illnesses. I gave you information in some detail about colds, flues, stomach flus, asthma, headaches, depression, stress, hypertension, allergies, diabetes, impotence, irritable bowel syndrome and fibromyalgia. I will continue to bring you other treatments for other illnesses in other volumes. But I do wish to give you a word of warning. Please do not get discouraged if the formula you are trying is not working for you. As with western medicine, traditional oriental medicine has many options to treat many illnesses. I have just attempted to bring you the most commonly used. But as every person is different, treatments are too and should be adapted to the individual. This is a subject that is well beyond the scope of this book and is covered substantially by authors such as Peter Deadman and John Chen.

As this book comes to an end, I want to leave you with the understanding that Oriental medicine is all about preventing illness. As such, I am going to give you simple tools you can use every day to improve your chances of successfully fighting an illness on your own. I goal is always to keep your body in balance.

Tips for healthy living

The first tip would be to stimulate ST36 every day. Tibetan monks often moxa this point during their meditation. How to use moxa should be learned before attempting to do it on oneself. It is a simple technique that I teach in my seminars regularly.

The second tip would be to stimulate the points on the back along the UB meridian. These points are associated with your organs, and stimulating them is like giving your internal tissues a mini massage, and thus a well-deserved energy boost.

Finally, the use of **Cordyceps** as a general regulator is highly recommended. To learn more about the mushroom, please read "Cordyceps:

treating diabetes, cancer and other illnesses". It is an easy read that will give you the understanding you need to make informed decisions about your health. The other formula that works wonders is "**Imperial tonic**" from Evergreen Herbs. I have seen it boost people with fatigue, and greatly improve their general health.

All that being said, nothing compares to consulting a health care professional who knows what he is talking about. Many illnesses are treatable at home. But a condition that lasts is a condition that possibly needs professional medical attention. Don't think this book can replace that. Should you have a difficult time finding the health care professional of your dreams, please feel free to contact my office at 818-230-2419 or email me directly at nvalkov@ttphc.com. We might be able to help.

One final word of caution: Pregnant women should consult a knowledgeable health care provider before attempting to self-medicate at home.